# A No-Fluff Guide to

# Pharmacy Calculations

A Step-by-Step simplified guide to master Pharmacy Calculations for Technicians

## CLEMENT

# CARTER

# Copyright

# Table of Contents

# Introduction

Assume you've just relocated to a new city and need to learn how to navigate. Would you prefer to be given a map or a comprehensive list of precise directions on how to travel between all of the city's various points? This book takes the position that learning to read a map once is simpler than memorizing several different instructions. You'll be able to swiftly set up and solve pharmaceutical calculation issues without the need for notes or formulae after learning a few fundamental ideas.

This guide will further reveal everything concerning solving pharmacy calculations especially for pharmacy technicians.

The following topics are covered:

- Rounding Numbers
- Numerals in Roman Numerals
- The System of Metrics
- The notation used in science
- Important Numbers
- Error Percentage
- The Household/Apothecary/Avoirdupois Systems

The most significant part is Dimensional Analysis and Ratio Proportion, which covers around 80% of the calculations encountered in pharmacy. One simple approach may be used to solve all of the issues in this chapter.

The following are some of the topics covered:

- Ratio Proportion vs. Dimensional Analysis
- Converting Units
- Calculations for Dosage
- Calculations for IV Flow Rates
- Calculations of percent/percent strength/ratio strength
- Calculations in milliequivalents

The following is a glossary of terms used in this book:

- Number: Integers, decimal numbers, and fractions are all included in this category.
- All positive and negative whole numbers, as well as zero, are integers.
- -4, -3, 0, 2, 25 are some examples.
- A number with a decimal point is called a decimal number.
- 25.3, 0.05, and so on are some examples.
- Fraction: A number expressed as a/b, where a and b are both integers, but b cannot be 0.
- 1/2, 3/4, 7/8, -1/2 are some examples.
- Unit: A measuring unit. Examples include milligrams, milliliters, kilograms, and liters.

A Few Points to Keep in Mind:

- Always include all units of measurement in your calculations (mg, g, L, mL, and so on). The most significant aspect of the computation is the units. The figures are just along for the trip.

- Make sure the computations are right mathematically. 0.25 X 100 percent equals 25%, not 0.25 X 100 percent equals 25%.
- Separate the number and the unit by a space. 5 mL (not 5 mL)
- When writing decimal values smaller than one, always use leading zeros. Not.5 mg, but 0.5 mg.
- Trailing zeros should never be used after entire numbers. Not 5.0 mg, but 5 mg
- Use mcg instead of g for micrograms, since g might be confused with mg.
- The scope of the definitions in this guide is confined to pharmacy practice. Electrolytes are ions that are crucial to the body's operation, but you won't obtain a thorough technical description.

# Chapter 1

# Essential Skills

## The Metric System

In pharmacy, the metric system is the most often used measuring system. Also, in pharmacy, the gram, liter, and meter are the most used basic units. Each of the foundation units may be multiplied or divided by ten to create bigger or smaller units.

Prefixes are used to distinguish between bigger and smaller units before the base units. The most often used metric units in pharmacy are included in the first table below.

## The Metric System Basics for Pharmacy Technicians

| Prefix | Symbol | Multiple of base | Weight | Volume | Length |
|--------|--------|------------------|--------|--------|--------|
| micro | mc | 1/1,000,000 | mcg | | |
| mili | m | 1/1000 | mg | mL | mm |
| centi | c | 1/100 | | | cm |
| | | Base Unit | g (gram) | L (liter) | m (meter) |
| kilo | k | 1000 | kg | | km |

4

# Approximate Equivalents to Selected Metric Units

| Weight Unit | Approximate Equivalent | Volume Unit | Approximate Equivalent | Length Unit | Approximate Equivalent |
|---|---|---|---|---|---|
| mcg | 1 ant leg? | mL | 20 drops | mm | 1/25 inch |
| mg | 6 grains of salt | L | 1 quart | cm | 4/10 inch |
| g | 1 paperclip | | | m | 1 yard |
| kg | 2.2 lb | | | km | 6/10 mile |

# Metric Prefixes Between $10^{18}$ and $10^{-18}$

| Prefix | Symbol | Multiplication Factor | Exponent |
|---|---|---|---|
| exa | E | 1000000000000000000 | $10^{18}$ |
| Peta | P | 1000000000000000 | $10^{15}$ |
| tera | T | 1000000000000 | $10^{12}$ |
| Giga | G | 1000000000 | $10^{9}$ |
| mega | M | 1000000 | $10^{6}$ |
| kilo | k | 1000 | $10^{3}$ |
| hector | h | 100 | $10^{2}$ |
| deca | da | 10 | $10^{1}$ |
| | Base Unit | 1 | $10^{0}$ |
| deci | d | 0.1 | $10^{-1}$ |

| centi | c | 0.01 | $10^{-2}$ |
|-------|---|------|-----------|
| milli | m | 0.001 | $10^{-3}$ |
| micro | mc | 0.000001 | $10^{-6}$ |
| nano | n | 0.000000001 | $10^{-9}$ |
| pico | p | 0.000000000001 | $10^{-12}$ |
| femto | f | 0.000000000000001 | $10^{-15}$ |
| atto | a | 0.000000000000000001 | $10^{-18}$ |

# Chapter 2

# Apothecary/Avoirdupois/ Household Systems

Although these systems are no longer widely used in pharmacy, there are a few units and critical elements that should be taught.

- **Weight Units:** Grain (gr): 64.8 mg technically, but generally rounded to 65 mg.

The ounce (oz) is a unit of measurement that is technically 28.3 g but is often rounded to 30 g.

- 16 ounces per pound (lb): The weight is usually rounded to 454 g.
- **Units of Volume:** Fluidram/fluid dram: 3.7 mL in technical terms, but commonly rounded up to 5 mL. Technically, a fluid ounce is 29.6 mL, although it's generally rounded up to 30 mL.
- A pint is equal to 16 fluid ounces. Technically, it's 473 milliliters, but it's generally rounded up to 480 milli-liters.
- 5 mL (teaspoonful)
- 15 mL/tablespoonful

## Significant Units with Rounded Metric Equivalents

| Apothecary Volume | Household Volume | Metric Volume |
|---|---|---|
| 1 fluidram /fluid dram | 1 teaspoonful (tsp) | 5 mL |
| 1 fluid ounce | 2 tablespoonfuls (tbs) | 30 mL |
| 16 fluid ounces | 1 pint (pt) | 480 mL (473 mL) |
| | 1 tablespoonful | 15 mL |
| **Apothecary Weight** | | **Metric Weight** |
| 1 grain (gr) | | 65 mg |
| | | |
| **Avoirdupois Weight** | **Household Weight** | **Metric Weight** |
| 1 ounce (oz) | 1 ounce (oz) | 30 g |
| 1 pound (lb) | 1 pound (lb) | 454 g |

*NB: Although these systems are not usually used currently, the records of these systems are exciting and can be seen online.*

# Ratios

## Tools Shed (Conversion Factors)

These conversion factors add up to 1 and maybe turned around if necessary. 1 g in metric weight

- 1000 mg  1 gram = 1 kilogram
- 1000 g  1 gram 1 milligram
- 1000 mcg 1 milligram
- 1 L (metric volume) 1000 mL
- 1 liter

- metric - 30 g in weight
- 1 oz
- 2.2 lb (30 g)
- 1 pound
- 1 pound 2.2 lb
- 454 g
- 1 pound
- 1 teaspoon metric 5 ml
- 1 tblsp 1 ounce
- 30 mL
- 1 oz 1 point
- 480 mL
- 1 tbsp 15 mL
- 1 tablespoon 1 tbsp
- 3 tbsp
- 16 ounces 1 tbsp
- 1 point
- 1 quart (16 oz)
- 8 oz. 2 pt.
- 1 cup
- 1 gallon (8 oz)
- 4 quarts 1 gallon
- 1 m in metric length
- 100 cm
- 1 meter 1 centimeter
- ten millimeters
- 1 centimeter

- 2.54 cm

## Metric Volume: 1 fl Dram Apothecary

- 5 mL
- 1 fl ounce 1 fl dram
- 30 mL
- 1 fluid ounce
- Metric Apothecary 65 milligrams in weight
- 1 gram 1 gram
- 65 micrograms

**Percentage: 1**

- 100 percent of the time
- 1st (100 percent )
- 60-second timer
- 1 minute
- 60 seconds 60 minutes
- 1 hour 1 hour
- 60 minutes 24 hours

# Dimensional Analysis and Ratio Proportion

**Dimensional Analysis (DA):** A strong approach for addressing issues in pharmacy, chemistry, physics, and engineering that involves multiplying a given by one or more ratios to achieve the solution.

Ratio Proportion (RP): A technique for comparing two ratios that are commonly utilized in the medical sector to address difficulties.

You must comprehend everything in this part completely:

The majority of computations in pharmacy simply entail adjusting the units from what is supplied to the units requested. These are some of them:

- Converting Units
- Dosage Calculations
- Calculations for IV Flow Rates
- Calculations for percent, percent strength, and ratio strength
- Calculations in milliequivalents

All of these computations may be done using DA or RP.

Consider them to be a single sort of computation using five distinct types of units, rather than five discrete types of calculations.

The three elements of each issue are the same:

- The Answer's Units: Think of it as the final destination.
- A Given: This is the starting point for the issue, and it is turned into the solution. • One or more Ratios: These are the instruments that are used to convert the provided units into the response units.

**Example 1: Convert 4.5 g to mg using DA.**

- The answer is in milligrams. This is where you'll arrive.
- The indicated weight is 4.5 grams. This is where it all begins.
- The weight-to-weight ratio is 1000 mg/g. This is the tool for converting grams to milligrams.
- Begin by writing down the beginning position and the final destination. This will aid in the placement of the ratio (s). mg = 4.5 g

Place the ratio with the answer units on top and the canceled units on the bottom. Multiply the provided by the ratio to get the answer. The grams cancel each other out, leaving mg in the solution.

**Example 2 with DA: A patient is given 400 mg of DA. The medication is available in a 200 mg/mL strength. How many milliliters will the patient drink?**

- The answer is given in milliliters (mL).
- The dose is 400 milligrams.
- It's a 200 mg/mL ratio.
- Begin by writing down the beginning position and the final destination, such as mL = 400 mg
- Arrange the ratio such that the answer units are at the top and the units to be canceled are at the bottom. Multiply the provided by the ratio to get the answer. The mg cancel each other out, leaving just mL.

- In this situation, the ratio was reversed, with mL at the top and mg at the bottom.

## The Ratios' Most Important Points

- The ratios are always one to one. Because 1000 mg equals 1 gram, 1000 mg
- 1 g = 1 (This form of ratio is used in this guide.)
- Because it is always true, it is referred to as an "off the shelf" ratio. A gram always contains 1000 mg.)

In example 2, the drug's strength is indicated to be 200 mg/mL. 1 mL = 200 mg is used to solve this issue. 1 milliliter

- 200 milligrams equal one milligram, and 200 milligrams equal one milli
- 1 milliliter equals one milliliter. (This sort of ratio is discussed in this book.)

Because it exclusively applies to the situation at hand, it's termed a "custom ratio." Only if the issue specifies 200 mg/mL will there be 200 mg/mL.)

- If necessary, the ratios may be turned upside down.

Following is an explanation of the ratio proportion technique.

Another approach used to answer the questions in this chapter is the ratio proportion method. The ratio proportion technique, also known as the ratio and proportion method, involves setting up two proportional (equal) ratios and solving for the unknown. Using the examples above as a guide:

**Example 1: Convert 4.5 g to mg using RP.**

- The RP technique employs two ratios: one for the unknown and one for the provided, with the latter functioning as a reference ratio.

The simplest technique to get x mg is to cross multiply (4.5 g)(1000 mg) and then divide by 1 g, yielding 4500 mg.

**Example 2 with RP: A patient is given 400 mg of RP. The medication is available in a 200 mg/mL strength. How many milliliters will the patient drink?**

- For x mL, multiply (400 mg)(1 mL)/200 mg = 2 mL

Both numerators and denominators must have the same units when utilizing the ratio proportion technique.

In terms of simplicity of use and safety, there isn't much of a difference between DA and RP for basic one-step issues. Consider the following issue, which is addressed using both DA and RP and includes numerous ratios.

**Example 3: A dose of 20 mg/kg has been given for a 186-pound patient. The medicine comes in 10 mL vials that each contain 2.5 g of the substance. How many milliliters should be given?**

- The answer is given in milliliters (mL).
- The weight is 186 pounds.
- The doses are 20 mg/kg, 2.5 g/10 mL, 2.2 lb/kg, and 1000 mg/g, respectively.

**Example 3 with RP: A 20 mg/kg dose has been given for a 186-pound patient. The medicine comes in 10 mL vials that each contain 2.5 g of the substance. How many milliliters should be given?**

- Step 1: Convert 186 pounds to kilograms. 84.5 kg is obtained by solving for x kg.
- Step 2: Determine the medicine dosage in milligrams for a patient weighing 84.5 kg. 1690 mg is obtained by solving for x mg.
- Step 3: Calculate 1690 mg in grams. 1.69 g is obtained by solving for x g.
- Step 4: Determine the mL dosage required to deliver 1.69 g of medication. 6.8 mL is the result of solving for x mL.

For situations requiring more than one step, the author believes that the dimensional analysis approach is preferable to the ratio proportion method.

- By canceling out the units before doing any computations, the issue may be built up in one step and evaluated for correctness using dimensional analysis. • When using the ratio proportion approach, numerous difficulties must be put up, which complicates the problem and introduces mistake sources.

- An "RP shovel" can move a small mound of gravel, but a "DA bulldozer" must be used to move a huge amount.

For easy unit conversion issues, both the DA and RP methods will be provided in the future, but only the DA approach will be shown for the other difficulties.

# Chapter 3

# Rounding Numbers

Calculated solutions often include more decimal places than necessary or intended, necessitating rounding. To round a number, first, identify the digit that will be rounded to. If you were requested to round to the closest tenth, you would look at the number 8 in the example below.

| 3 | 5 | 6 | . | 8 | 1 | 9 |
|---|---|---|---|---|---|---|
| Hundreds | Tens | Ones | Decimal Point | Tenths | Hundredths | Thousandths |

Look at the digit that comes after the digit that is being rounded.

- If the next digit is 0,1,2,3, or 4, all the digits after the rounded digit are discarded, and you're done. The 1 and 9 are removed in the previous example, leaving 356.8 as the rounded number.
- If the next digit is 5,6,7,8, or 9, all digits after the rounded digit are discarded, and the digit is increased by one. When rounding the number 156.879 to the closest tenth, the 7 and 9 are removed, and the 8 is raised to 9, yielding 156.9.

**IMPORTANT:** When rounding numbers, just look at the first digit following the rounded digit. All other numbers are meaningless.

Round to the closest tenth, for example:

- 6.8 is the rounded version of 6.759 (Look only at the 5; the 9 is irrelevant.)
- 10.248 is equal to 10.248 rounded up (Look only at the 4; the 8 is irrelevant.)
- 0.4 is 0.38999 rounded up. (Only look at the 8's; the 9's are unimportant.)

Round to the closest hundredth, for example:

- 89.52 is the rounded version of 89.523.

- 0.59788 equals 0.60 when rounded.
- 7.2395 is 7.24 when rounded.

# Scientific Notation

Scientific notation is a more convenient means of writing very big and extremely tiny numbers.

- For example, in scientific notation, 602,200,000,000,000,000,000,000 becomes 6.022 X 1023.
- For example, in scientific notation, 0.0000000000000-000019942 becomes 1.9942 X 10-18.

# Terminology

The little number written immediately above and to the right of a base number is called an exponent. It is the 23rd digit in 6.022 X 1023, and it represents the number of times 10 is multiplied. 10 X 10 is represented by the number 102. 10 X 10 X 10 is represented by the number 103.

A negative exponent signifies a number smaller than one when 1 is divided by tens. For instance, 102 is 1/102, or 1/100, or 0.01.

**Coefficient:** The result of multiplying a number by ten and raising it to the exponent. It's the 6.022 in the 6.022 X 1023 equation. It's always at least one and never more than ten.

# How to Write a Number in Scientific Notation Step-by-Step

Using 6,154,000,000 and 0.000816 as examples:

1. Separate the digits that are either before or after all of the zeros, then add a decimal point after the first digit to produce the coefficient.

- 6.154,000,000: 6.154,000,000,000,000,000,000,000,000,000,000,000,000,000,000,000,000,000,000,000,000,000,000,000,000,000
- 0.000816: 8.1616161616161616161616161616161616

2. Count the number of places to shift the decimal point from the coefficient's decimal point to the end or back to the original decimal point from the original integer.

- 6,154,000,000: 9 spots between 6 and 1 to the finish.
- 0.000816: 4 places back from the initial decimal point between 8 and 1.

3. Multiply the coefficient by 10 increased to the number of places the decimal point was shifted. The exponent is positive if the decimal point is moved to the right; it is negative if the decimal point is moved to the left.

- 6.154 X 109
- 8.16 X 10-4

| Number | Scientific Notation |
|---|---|
| 5,015,000 | $5.015 \times 10^6$ |
| 3,000 | $3 \times 10^3$ |
| 645,000,000 | $6.45 \times 10^8$ |
| 0.00056 | $5.6 \times 10^{-4}$ |
| 0.00000734 | $7.34 \times 10^{-6}$ |
| 0.00003005 | $3.005 \times 10^{-5}$ |

# Significant Figures

In the world, there are two sorts of numbers: precise and inexact. Exact: 5 + 7 equals 35. The result of 1 divided by 4 is 0.25.

All measurements are approximate. (Note that counting is not the same as measuring). When a measurement is taken, the findings are provided as a number that indicates the measurement's accuracy. The digits that indicate the measurement's precision are deemed to be important.

For example, since the line was obviously over the 3 cm mark and nearly halfway to the 4 cm mark, a line measured with a ruler marked off in centimeters may be reported as 3.5 cm. There are two major figures in this measurement. If the same line is measured with an mm-marked ruler and the line is found to be approximately halfway between the 6 mm and

7 mm marks of the fourth cm, the measurement is reported as 3.65 cm. There are three key figures in this measurement.

- Consider significant numbers to be a message from the person who measured the people reading it, indicating the measurement's correctness. A measurement of 1.015 kg, for example, represents an extremely precise measurement, but a measurement of 1 kg does not.
- Measurements include all digits that are known to be precise, as well as one digit that is an approximation.

## Rules for Significant Figures

1.  All numbers that are not zero are significant. The numbers 1,2,3,4,5,6,7,8,9 are all crucial. There are seven major digits in 67825.98.

2.  Between two nonzero values, all zeros are important. There are five major figures in the number 57801.

3.  Leading zeros have no bearing. Small decimal values, such as 0.000512, have leading zeros (zeros in front). The zero before the decimal and the three zeros after the decimal are unimportant since their main function is to keep the places straight. There are three important numbers in 0.000512.

4.  If the number has a decimal point, the trailing zeros are important. The two zeros at the end were included

merely to express the fact that the measurement was exact to the hundredth place, therefore 856.00 includes five significant numbers.

5.     Trailing zeros in a number without a decimal point are usually unimportant. There are two key numbers in the number 25,000. Writing 25,000 in scientific notation as 2.5000 x 104, which now includes five significant digits, is the greatest way to convey it to one spot.

## The Simplest Way to Summarize the Rules:

Is there a decimal point in the number? If the answer is yes, then all of the statistics are meaningful.

Except for the zeros in front, the first digit is not zero. 0,00579,00000 (6 significant figures)

## Examples:

If the answer is no, then all figures are incorrect.

Except for the zeros following the final nonzero digit, none of the numbers are important.

| Number | # of Significant Figures |
|---|---|
| 506 | 3 |
| 450 | 2 |
| 5645 | 4 |
| 0.00051 | 2 |
| 5.1070 | 5 |
| 0.25 | 2 |
| 5600 | 2 |
| 5600.0 | 5 |
| 980005 | 6 |
| 980000 | 2 |
| 0.00050 | 2 |
| $6.7500 \times 10^4$ | 5 |

# Significant Figures Adding and Subtracting Rules

If the units are the same, the sum or difference of two or more measures containing significant numbers may only include as many decimal places as the measurement with the least number of decimal places.

14.151 mg + 3.2 mg = 17.351 mg, for example:

- The number of decimal places in 3.2 mg is the smallest: one.

The answer must be rounded to the nearest tenth of a milligram: 17.4 mg.

# Significant Figures Multiplication and Division Rules

- When multiplying or dividing two measures with significant figures, the outcome can only have the same amount of significant figures as the measurement with the fewest significant figures.

Example: $(3,881.4 \text{ m2}) = (1.5 \text{ m})(2587.6 \text{ m})$.

- The number of significant figures in 1.5 m is the smallest: two.
- 3,900 m2 is the result, which must be rounded to two significant numbers.

# Roman Numerals

The Arabic number system, often known as the decimal number system, is a positional number system in which the value of a digit is determined by its location. The 2 in 521 is equal to 20, yet the 2 in 245 is equal to 200.

The Roman numeral system is an additive and subtractive system with a fixed value for each numeral. The C in CXX, like the C in CLXV, denotes a value of 100.

# Roman Numerals and Their Values

| Roman Numeral | Value | Memory Hints |
|---|---|---|
| SS | 1/2 | Short stack of pancakes, which is about half a regular stack. |
| I | 1 | Easy to remember because it looks like a 1. |
| V | 5 | Your hand with your fingers together and thumb apart forms a V. |
| X | 10 | Think of it as two V's, one on top of the other. |
| L | 50 | Think of Lasso. It has 5 letters and ends in O (50). |
| C | 100 | Think of Century or C-note. |
| D | 500 | Imagine 500 Dogs in your house, all barking and running around. |
| M | 1000 | Think of Millennium. |

# Forming Roman Numerals Rules

1. Begin on the left with the greatest number and work your way to the right with the smallest. 2) No more than three consecutive numbers must be the same. XXXX cannot be written as 40.

2. When a smaller number precedes a bigger number, the smaller number is deducted from the larger number. For instance, IV equals 4 when the I is removed from V. (5-1).

3. Only the letters I, X, and C are allowed to be deducted from a greater number. A greater number cannot be deducted from the "five" numerals (V, L, D). The number 45 is written as XLV, not VL.

5.  When subtracting a smaller number from a bigger numeral, the smaller numeral must be at least one-tenth of the larger numeral. IX is 9, however, IL and IC are not allowed for 49 or 99. XLIX is the code for 49, while XCIX is the code for 99. Only one digit may be removed at a time, and from only one other numeral. IX X is not allowed for 8, and IIXX is not allowed for 19.

6.  Always use the biggest possible numbers. Even though writing three V's does not violate rule #2, 15 is written XV, not VVV.

These principles may seem difficult, but with a little practice and the accompanying advice, Roman numerals will become second nature.

- Only if the number includes a 4 or 9 must a smaller numeral be subtracted from a bigger numeral. 246 is written CCXLVI, with the X deducted from the L. 2386 is written MMCCCLXXXXVI, with no subtraction.
- When subtracting one number from another, consider them as a unit. Consider IV as 4, not 5-1, XL as 40, not 50-10, and so on.

# Check the following table to be able to quickly form any Roman numeral

| 1000 | M | 100 | C | 10 | X | 1 | I |
|------|-----|-----|------|----|------|-----|------|
| 2000 | MM | 200 | CC | 20 | XX | 2 | II |
| 3000 | MMM | 300 | CCC | 30 | XXX | 3 | III |
| | | 400 | CD | 40 | XL | 4 | IV |
| | | 500 | D | 50 | L | 5 | V |
| | | 600 | DC | 60 | LX | 6 | VI |
| | | 700 | DCC | 70 | LXX | 7 | VII |
| | | 800 | DCCC | 80 | LXXX | 8 | VIII |
| | | 900 | CM | 90 | XC | 9 | IX |
| | | | | | | 1/2 | SS |

## Example: Convert 2648 to a Roman number

- Separate the 1000s, 100s, 10s, and 1s and label them with the appropriate Roman number.

| | |
|---|---|
| 2000 | MM |
| 600 | DC |
| 40 | XL |
| 8 | VIII |

Arrange the Roman numerals in ascending order, beginning with the biggest. MMDCXLVIII\s8

## Example of Auxiliary Subjects for Pharmacy Technicians Calculations: Convert MCMXXXIV to a number.

- Split the 1000s, 100s, 10s, and 1s and write the relevant number next to each one.

| | |
|---|---|
| M | 1000 |
| CM | 900 |
| XXX | 30 |
| IV | 4 |

# Chapter 3

## Unit Conversions

- **Unit:** A metric of measurement. The units of measurement used in pharmacy calculations are milligrams, grams, milliliters.
- **Unit Conversions:** Impacting the value of one unit without changing the value of another.

The "Tool Shed," so named because it includes the tools necessary to transform the provided units into the desired units, is included in this section.

## How to Use the DA Method's Tools

- On the left side of the equation, write down the amount to be translated, such as 8.67 g, and on the right side of the equation, write down the units of the response, such as mg. mg = 8.67 g
- Look for the tool (the conversion factor) with mg on top and g on the bottom in the tool shed. 1000 mg may be found under Metric Weight.
- Next to the amount to be converted, place the tool to be used, cancel out the units, and multiply.
- More than one tool may be required to complete the conversion. Consider the following scenario: In 3.5 meters, how many inches are there?

# How to Use the RP Method's Tools

- Write a ratio with x at the top, the answer's units at the bottom, and the provided at the top. Using the 8.67 g to mg conversion as an example:

- In the tool shed, find a ratio with mg on top and g on the bottom. This is the reference ratio against which the unknown ratio will be compared. Between them, put an equal symbol.

- Divide by 1 g to get x mg (8.67 g)(1000 mg). x mg = 8670 mg • If more than one tool is required, create a new issue with the first solution as the supplied answer, or use the DA technique instead.

# Converting Units in the Metric System

| Metric Measurements | | |
|---|---|---|
| **Length** | **Mass** | **Volume/Capacity** |
| 1 kilometer (km) = 1000 m | 1 kilogram (kg) = 1000 g | 1 kiloliter (kL) = 1000 L |
| 1 hectometer (hm) = 100 m | 1 hectogram (hg) = 100 g | 1 hectoliter (hL) = 100 L |
| 1 dekameter (dam) = 10 m | 1 dekagram (dag) = 10 g | 1 dekaliter (daL) = 10 L |
| 1 meter (m) = 1 m | 1 gram (g) = 1 g | 1 liter (L) = 1 L |
| 1 decimeter (dm) = 0.1 m | 1 decigram (dg) = 0.1 g | 1 deciliter (dL) = 0.1 L |
| 1 centimeter (cm) = 0.01 m | 1 centigram (cg) = 0.01 g | 1 centiliter (cL) = 0.01 L |
| 1 millimeter (mm) = 0.001 m | 1 milligram (mg) = 0.001 g | 1 milliliter (mL) = 0.001 L |
| 1 meter = 100 centimeters | 1 gram = 100 centigrams | 1 liter = 100 centiliters |
| 1 meter = 1000 millimeters | 1 gram = 1000 milligrams | 1 liter = 1000 milliliters |

Units in the metric system are connected by powers of two. Their names' fundamental words indicate this relationship. A meter, for example, is the most fundamental unit for measuring length. One kilometer is equal to 1000

The prefix kilo- denotes a thousand. A centimeter is a unit of measurement. 1/100 centimeters, since the word centi- denotes one-hundredth of a meter (just as one cent denotes one-hundredth of a meter). The metric system's measurement equivalencies are presented in the reference table below. In parenthesis, you'll find the standard acronyms for each measurement.

We'll use the same method for conversions in the metric system as we did in the US system. To get to the right units, we'll multiply by a conversion factor of one using the identity feature of multiplication.

Have you ever participated in a 5k or 10k race? The distances between the start and finish lines are measured in kilometers. When discussing the duration of a race in the United States, the metric system is often employed.

**Example**

**John completed a ten-kilometer race. What was the distance he covered?**

## Answer:

The kilometer will be converted to meters with the identity property of multiplication as well as the equivalencies in the reference table from the previous table.

| | |
|---|---|
| | 10 kilometers |
| Multiply the measurement to be converted by 1. | $10km \cdot 1$ |
| Write 1 as a fraction relating kilometers and meters. | $10km \cdot \frac{1000m}{1km}$ |
| Simplify. | $\frac{10km \cdot 1000m}{1km}$ |
| Multiply. | $10,000$ m |
| | Nick ran $10,000$ meters. |

# Household, Apothecary, and Metric Unit Conversions

## Measurement Techniques

## PART A - Conversions in One Step

We can convert from one measuring system to another using a straight conversion factor.

## Conversion Table

| Mass | Volume | Length | Time |
|---|---|---|---|
| 1 g = 1000 mg | 1 tsp = 5 mL | 1 inch = 2.5 cm | 1 h = 60 min |
| 1 mg = 1000 mcg | 1 tbsp = 3 tsp (15 mL) | 12 inches = 1 foot | 1 minute = 60 |
| 1 oz = 30 g | 2 tbsp = 1 fluid oz | 100 cm = 1 meter | seconds |
| 1 lb = 16 oz | 1 cup = 8 oz | 1000 m = 1 km | 1 day = 24 hours |
| 1 lb= 454 g | 1 cup = 250 mL | 1 yard = 3 feet | 1 week = 7 days |
| 2.2 lb = 1 kg | 1 L = 1000 mL | 1 mile = 1.6 km | 1 year = 12 |
| 1 kg = 1000 g | 1 pint = 2 cups | | months |
| 1 metric ton = 1000 kg | 1 quart = 2 pints | | 1 year = 365 |
| | 1 gallon = 4 quarts | | days |

**Conversion Rules**

1. Multiply the beginning measurement by the conversion factor when converting from a LARGER to a SMALLER unit. For instance, 1 meter equals 100 centimeters. Because a meter is LARGER than a yardstick, multiplied by the centimeter 1 cm (conversion factor 100).
2. Divide the beginning measurement by the conversion factor when going from a SMALLER to a LARGER unit. 1000 milliliters = 1 liter 1000 Because a milliliter is a fraction of a liter, L1 mL is multiplication by the conversion factor (1000).

# Apothecary, household, and metric measurement systems

**For instance: Convert 5 cups to mL**

1. Determine the conversion factor between our initial measurement and the unit we want to use. We can see from our conversion table that 1 cup equals 250 mL.
2. Multiply the initial measurement by the conversion factor and simplify since we're going from a LARGER to a SMALLER unit. As a result, 5 cups contain 1250 mL.

**Example 2: Convert 154 pounds to kilograms.**

1. Determine the conversion factor between our initial measurement and the unit we want to use. We can see from our conversion table that 2.2 lb Equals 1 kilogram.

2. Divide the initial measurement by the conversion factor and simplify since we're going from a SMALLER to a LARGER unit. Thus, in 154 lb, there is 70 kg.

# Conversions in Multiple Steps

We may not have a straight conversion factor in certain circumstances. We must combine many conversions to convert from one unit of measure to another.

**Another Example: Convert 65 into m.**

1. Determine the conversion factor between our initial measurement and the unit we want to use. We'll divide the conversion into two phases since there isn't a straight translation from into m. a) inch cm; b) cm m; c) cm m; d) cm m; e

2. Our conversion factor for portion a) is 1 in = 2.5 cm. Multiply the initial measurement by the conversion factor and simplify since we're going from a LARGER to a SMALLER unit.

3. Our conversion factor for section b) is 100 cm = 1 m. Divide the initial measurement by the conversion factor

and simplify since we're going from a SMALLER to a LARGER unit. In 65 in, there are 1.625 m.

**More Examples: Convert 5.2 L to tsp.**

1. Determine the conversion factor between our initial measurement and the unit we want to use. We'll divide the conversion into two sections since there isn't a simple translation from L to tsp. a) mL tsp; b) mL tsp; c) mL tsp; d) mL t.
2. Our conversion factor in section a) is 1 L = 1000 mL. Multiply the initial measurement by the conversion factor and simplify since we're going from a LARGER to a SMALLER unit.
3. Our conversion factor for component b) is 5 mL = 1 tsp. Divide the initial measurement by the conversion factor and simplify since we're going from a SMALLER to a LARGER unit. In 5.2 L, there is 1040 tsp.

**NOTE:** There are alternative ways to translate between different measuring systems. Alternative approaches may be found in the TLC handouts "Dimensional Analysis" and "Conversions in the Metric System."

Convert between the apothecary, domestic, and metric measuring systems in this exercise.

1) 4 tsp (into mL) =

2) 5 oz (into g) =

3) $2\frac{3}{5}$ cups (into mL) =

4) 400 mL (into L ) =

5) 8 tbsp (into ml) =

6) 450 g (into oz) =

7) 12 in (into cm) =

8) 200 lb (into kg) =

9) 197 in (into m) =

10) 650 mL (into cups) =

11) 30 ml (into tbsp.) =

12) 5 kg (into lb) =

13) 3 m (into in) =

14) 5 tbsp (into fluid oz ) =

15) 5 feet 3 in (into m ) =

16) 5 m (into feet and inches) =

17) 5.2 L (into tsp) =

18) 1600 mg (into oz) =

19) 60 mL (into tbsp) =

20) $2\frac{2}{5}$ tbsp (into tsp) =

## Solutions:

1) **20 mL** (1 tsp = 5 mL)

2) **150 g** (1 oz = 30 g)

3) **650 mL** (1 cup = 250 mL)

4) **0.4 L** (1000 mL = 1 L)

5) **120 mL** (1 tbsp = 15 mL)

6) **15 oz** (30 g = 1 oz)

7) **30 cm** (1inch = 2.5 cm)

8) **90.9 kg** (2.2 lb = 1 kg)

9) **4.925 m** (1 inch = 2.5 cm; 100 cm = 1 m)

10) **2.6 cups** (250 mL = 1 cup)

11) **2 tbsp** (15 mL = 1 tbsp)

12) **11 lb** (1 kg = 2.2 lb)

13) **300 cm = 120 in** (2.5 cm = 1 inch)

14) **2.5 fluid oz** (2 tbsp = 1 fluid oz)

15) **63 inches = 157.5 cm = 1.575 m** (1 foot = 12 inches; 1 inch = 2.5 cm)

16) **500 cm = 200 inches = 16'8"** (1 m = 100 cm; 2.5 cm = 1 inch; 12 inches = 1 foot)

17) **5200 mL = 1040 tsp** (1L = 1000 mL; 5 mL = 1 tsp)

18) **1.6 g = 0.053 oz** (1000 mg = 1 g; 30 g = 1 oz)

19) **4 tbsp** (15 mL = 1 tbsp)

20) **$7\frac{1}{5}$ tsp** (1 tbsp = 3 tsp)

# Chapter 4

# Dosage Calculations

**Terminology:**

- **Dose:** The amount of medication given at one time.
- **Dosage:** The dosage information, as well as any other relevant information about the dose's frequency, duration, mode of administration, and so on.

For example, a patient is given 500 mg three times a day orally for ten days. The dose is 500 mg, taken three times a day for ten days.

- **mg/kg/day:** Amount of medicine supplied per kilogram of body weight per day in milligrams. mg/kg day is a theoretically comparable unit of measurement that is simpler to work within computations.

**Step 1:** Carefully read the issue, searching for the following three elements:

- **The Answer's Units:** The issue can ask, "How many mL, pills, mg, teaspoonfuls, or other units would the patient take?" Or you may state something more general, like What is weight, volume, and amount of suspension will be required?

- **The Problem's Given:** The problem may state, "A prescription is written for 10 mg, 20 mL, 1 g, and so on," or "A patient is to get 250 mg, 5 mL, and so on." • One or More Ratios: Every issue (apart from basic unit conversions) will include a ratio; all you have to do is learn to detect it. It might be 250 mg per 5 mL, 50 mg pill, 400 mcg per mL, or 3 g per 100 mL. To finish the computation, "off the shelf" ratios may be necessary.

**Step 2:** The following equation may be used to answer all of the issues using DA: • (Given)(Ratio 1)(Ratios 2, 3,... if necessary) =

The issue can be set up and addressed after the three components have been recognized.

For example, a patient will be given 500 mg of amoxicillin. A bottle of amoxicillin 250 mg/5mL suspension is available at the drugstore. How many milliliters of the suspension will be given to the patient at each dose?

- The answer is given in milliliters (mL).
- The dosage: 500mg
- The dosage is 250 mg
- 5 milliliters

**Step 3:** Now you may set up the problem:

- Use an equal sign to separate the provided and the units of the response. mL = 500 mg

- The ratio is the instrument that will be utilized to convert the provided units (mg) into the response units (mL). Remember that the ratios always equal 1 and can be turned around if necessary. The ratio must be set up such that the provided units are wiped out, leaving just the response units. The ratio must be switched in this situation, with mL on top and mg on the bottom.

# IV Flow Rate Calculations

These tasks seem to be stressful, yet there is no new arithmetic involved; simply new units, ratios, and language.

**Terminology:**

- **IV:** Abbreviation for intravenous, which means given via a vein.
- **Drop factor:** The number of drops per milliliter (gtts). Micro drip tubing has a density of 10, 15, and 20 gtts/mL, while micro drip tubing has a density of 60 gtts/mL.
- **Flow rate, infusion rate, or drip rate:** The amount of fluid or medicine supplied over time. Typically, the units are gtts/min, mL/hour, or mg/hour.

These issues are dealt with in the same way as unit conversion and dose issues are. There is a given unit of the response and one or more ratios that will be used to convert the given units to the answer's units. The key distinction is that the supply is generally a rate, therefore the given will have two units and the response will have two units.

**Example: A 50 mL/h IV with a drop factor of 15 (15 gtts/mL) is being administered. What is the gtts/min rate?**

- The supplied quantity is 50 mL and must be transformed into gtts
- Gtts must be converted from mL.

The drop factor of 15 drops was used to convert mL to gtts.

- Converting hours to minutes is required.
- The 60-minute ratio is used to convert hours to minutes.
- It's simplest to start by writing down the supplied and response units, then filling in the ratios, which may need to be flipped.
- First, insert the drop factor to convert mL to gtts.

# Percent and Ratio Strength Calculations

## Percent

The three main elements in comprehending % are: • Percentage refers to the number of times a number is multiplied by 100. 50 percent is equal to 50 parts per 100, or 50 percent.

- One hundred percent equals one. Because one hundred percent equals one, the conversion factors are 100 percent.

100 percent is equivalent to multiplying or dividing by 100 percent.

- Just like the units of measurement cancel themselves out, the percent sign (percent) will cancel itself out.

# How to Convert a Number to a Percentage

- Multiply a number by 100 percent to convert it to a percent.
- Convert 0.30 to a percentage, for example. 0.30 (one hundred percent) equals thirty percent. Because 100 percent equals 1, the value of 0.30 has remained the same; just the appearance has altered. How to Convert a Percentage to a Number
- Divide a percentage by 100 percent to get a number. You can multiply by if you want to.

# How to Convert a Fraction to a Percentage

- Multiply a fraction by 100 percent to convert it to a percentage.
- Convert 1/4 to a percent as an example. a quarter of a percent of a percent of a percent of a percent of a percent

**To summarize:** Multiply by 100 percent to add the percent symbol. Divide by 100 percent to get rid of the percent marker. (Yes, you multiply or divide by 100%, not 100 percent). Convert the following numbers to percent.

| Number | Percent |
|--------|---------|
| 0.87 | 0.87 (100%) = 87% |
| 1.67 | 1.67 (100%) = 167% |
| 0.0056 | 0.0056 (100%) = 0.56% |
| 0.36 | 0.36 (100%) = 36% |
| 3 | 3 (100%) = 300% |
| 1.1 | 1.1 (100%) = 110% |
| 0.9944 | 0.9944 (100%) = 99.44% |

## Convert the following percent to numbers

| Percent | Number |
|---------|--------|
| 89% | 89%/100% = 0.89 |
| 0.25% | 0.25%/100% = 0.0025 |
| 157% | 157%/100% = 1.57 |
| 99.44% | 99.44%/100% = 0.9944 |
| 56.1% | 56.1%/100% = 0.561 |
| 25% | 25%/100% = 0.25 |
| 34% | 34%/100% = 0.34 |

**Convert the following fractions to percentages.**

| Fraction | Percent |
| --- | --- |
| 5/6 | 5/6 (100%) = 83.3% |
| 9/10 | 9/10 (100%) = 90% |
| 2/20 | 2/20 (100%) = 10% |
| 1/4 | 1/4 (100%) = 25% |
| 34/50 | 34/50 (100%) = 68% |
| 2/8 | 2/8 (100%) = 25% |
| 13/99 | 13/99 (100%) = 13.1% |

# Percent Strength

The sole distinction between percent strength and % strength is that percent strength contains weight and volume measures.

- In a percent strength, weight is always stated in gram units (g). • In a percent strength, volume is always indicated in milliliters (mL).

**The Four Different Types of Mixtures (also Known as Solutions)**

- 1 g of hydrocortisone (the solute) in 100 g of finished cream is an example of weight in weight (the solution).

This is a hydrocortisone cream with a concentration of 1%.

- 1 g of NaCl (the solute) in 100 mL of NaCl solution is an example of weight in volume (the solution). This is a NaCl solution with a concentration of 1%.
- 1 mL of ethanol (the solute) in 100 mL of the end product (the solution) is an example of volume in volume (1 mL ethanol mixed with 99 mL of water). This is an ethanol solution with a concentration of 1%. This sort of solution is not particularly frequent in terms of volume in weight. 10 mL glycerin in 100 g glycerin ointment is an example. This is a glycerin ointment that contains 10% glycerin.
- A 1% NaCl solution is equal to 1% of NaCl solution. The units ww,wv,vv, and vw are sometimes not included in the problem and must be added. It is w if it is weighed, and v if it is measured in volume. It's worth noting that liquids are sometimes stated in weight.

## The Secret to Solving These Issues

- In the ratios and units of the solution, substitute g for w and mL for v. • Carry out the computations ahead of time.
- If necessary, return w and v to the final solution. For example, how many grams of NaCl are in 45 mL of a percent solution?

- This is an issue that can be solved in a single step. Replace w and v with g and mL, multiply by 45 mL, then divide by 100 percent.

See how well mL and percent cancel each other out? If the issue called for several milligrams, multiply it by 1000 milligrams.

## Calculate the Percent Strength by multiplying the weight and volume together

Set up the problem using the supplied and the answer's units to calculate the percent strength of a solution. The solution will be expressed in percent w/v, percent w/w, percent v/v, or percent v/w, but instead of w and v, g and mL will be used.

**Example:** If there are 985 mg of NaCl in 2.5 L, what is the percent strength of the solution?

- Write down the following information as well as the answer's units:

It's clear that mg has to be converted to g, L needs to be translated to mL, and the percent needs to be added.

- To convert mg to g, multiply by one gram. 1000 milligrams
- Multiply 1 L by L to convert L to mL. 1000 milliliters
- Multiply by 100 percent to add the percent symbol.
- In the final solution, substitute w for g and v for mL.

# Percent Error

A weight measurement mistake of 5 grams might indicate either an accurate or an erroneous measurement. A 5 g mistake weighing out 16 g of active ingredient for a prescription suggests an imprecise measurement with a big percent error, but a 5 g error weighing out a bag of potatoes denotes a very accurate measurement with a tiny percent error. It's critical to comprehend % error and know how to compute it.

**Terminology:**

- **Desired quantity:** The amount that is being attempted to be measured. Consider it the objective.
- **Measured quantity:** The amount that was measured.
- **Error quantity:** The absolute difference between the intended and actual amount. (A positive number is always used.)
- **Percent error:** The number of mistakes is represented as a percentage of the target amount. Percent Error Calculation

For example, you attempted to weigh a quantity of 100 g but discovered that you weighed 95 g.

- 100 g is the desired amount.
- The actual weight is 95 g.
- The amount of error is 5 g.

- Percentage error: 5% 5 percent of 100 g is 100 g.

**Important:** When calculating % error, always use the intended amount. For instance: The preferred weight is 525 g, but you weighed out 501 g.

| Desired Quantity (Target) | Actual Quantity | Error Quantity | Percent Error |
|---|---|---|---|
| 525 g | 501 g | 24 g | $\frac{24\,g}{525\,g} \times 100\% = 4.6\%$ |

# Ratio Strength

- Drug strengths are sometimes given as ratio strengths, which are equivalent to % strength estimates. The units are always grams and milliliters. w/w, w/v, v/v, or v/w solutions are possible.
- The standard format is 1: another number, where the other number represents the ultimate product quantity. 1:100, 1:500, and 1:10,000 are some examples.

- A 1:100 w/w formulation has 1 gram of active ingredient per 100 grams of the finished product. It's not 1 gram of active substance and 100 gram of inactive ingredient.
- 1 g active component in 100 mL solution is a 1:100 w/v solution.
- In a 1:100 v/v solution, 1 mL of the active component is present in 100 mL of solution.

- One mL of the active ingredient in 100 g of the product equals a 1:100 v/w solution.

# Instructions for relative strength calculations

- Determine the solution type (w/w, w/v, v/v, v/w).
- Assign the units of g and mL to w and v, respectively.
- Convert from the colon to the fraction format while keeping the units. For example, a ratio of 1:1000 w/v equals 1 g/1000 mL.

**Carry on with the computations using DA or RP**

Example: How much epinephrine is in 45 mL of a 1:10,000 epinephrine solution?

- This is a w (mg) epinephrine solution in v (45 mL).
- 1 g:10,000 mL (1:10,000 w/v)
- 1 g:10,000 mL equals 1 g when translated to fraction format. 10,000 milliliters
- Use DA to complete the computations.

- ✓ 1 gram 45 mL
- ✓ 1000 mg 10,000 mL
- ✓ 4.5 mg Equals 1 gram

**Important:** Many people have died resulting from improper ratio strength estimations, with epinephrine being one of the most prevalent medicines implicated. When calculating relative strength, use extreme caution. The strength of most medications labeled with a ratio strength will be indicated in mg/mL, which is safer to use.

# Chapter 5

# Concentration/Dilutions/Reconstitution Calculations

Calculations involving concentrations, dilution, and mixing are covered in this chapter. In this chapter, there are various distinct sorts of issues, yet they all contain similar components.

## The Alignment Method

When constructing a third strength, this approach is used to determine the volumes of two distinct strength solutions. It may also be utilized to solve certain smaller issues.

## Making a solution with two different strengths

The allegation approach covers this subject.

- Constructing a Solution Using a Diluent and a Stock Solution

The most typical sort of dilution calculation found in the pharmacy is this one. Several approaches to addressing these issues will be discussed.

- Calculating a Mixture's Percent Strength

These calculations seem to be difficult at first, but they are rather simple.

- Calculating Powder Volume

Mixing a diluent with a dry powder containing the active component is required for these calculations. These computations may or may not appear in your practice.

- Dilution in Sequence

The procedure for making an extremely dilute solution will be described.

# The Alignment Technique

- The alligation approach is a simple problem-solving technique that involves combining two separate strength solutions to create the third strength.
- Although it is not the most convenient way for tackling small dilution issues, it may be utilized if required.
- All strengths must be expressed as a percentage.

**Example: To make 1000 mL of a 22 percent solution, how much of a 10% solution must be combined with a 25% solution?**

**Step 1:** Draw a box and label the bottom left corner with the percent of the lower strength solution, the upper left corner with the percent of the higher strength solution, and the center with the percent of the solution is prepared. A 10 is put in the lower-left corner, a 25 in the upper left corner, and a 22 in the center in the illustration above.

**Step 2:** In the upper right corner, but the difference between the bottom left and center corners. Make a note of the difference between the upper left and center corners in the lower right corner. It's worth noting that the differences are always expressed as positive figures.

**Step 3:** The 12 and 3 reflect the number of components required to produce the 22 percent solution from the 25 percent solution and the 10% solution. Both solutions have a total of 15 parts (12 + 3), hence 12/15 of the final solution is the 25% solution, and 3/15 of the final solution is the 10% solution. To get the quantity of 25% solution, multiply 1000 mL by 12/15. To calculate the quantity of 10% solution to add, multiply 1000 mL by 3/15.

If the stock solution and end product are both specified in percent strength, this approach may also be used to make a solution from a stock solution and a diluent. Use a 0 in the lower-left corner and the default solution's percent strength in the upper left corner.

This is perhaps the most prevalent dilution issue found in pharmacies. There are three typical approaches to solve these issues:

- Determine the number of active components in the finished product, then figure out how much stock solution is needed to get the active ingredient.
- Use the formula V1C1=V2C2, where V1 represents the volume of the first solution, C1 represents the concentration of the first solution, V2 represents the volume of the second solution, and C2 represents the concentration of the second solution.
- Use the alligation approach, which is not the most convenient or time-saving option.

Consider the following problem, which was addressed using all three ways.

**A customer requests 600 mL of a 25 mg/mL solution. You have a stock solution of 100 mg/mL on hand. How many milliliters of the stock solution and milliliters of the diluent are required?**

Consider what Baker Bob did in a comparable scenario before looking at the three approaches. Bob got a big order for 600 birthday cakes with 25 candles apiece. "I'm preparing 600 cakes, and each cake will have 25 candles," he thought to himself, eager to purchase the ingredients for the cakes. "600 cakes multiplied by 25 candles each cake equals 15,000 candles." Bob next calls the candle distributor and inquires about the number of candles in a box. He's been informed that each package contains 100 candles. "I need 15,000 candles," Bob muses, "and they come 100 to a box." Bob then places an order for 150 boxes.

Bob didn't care what size box the candles came in until he added up the total number of candles; he didn't require a "candle formula."

**Method 1:** Determine the number of active components in the finished product, then determine the volume of stock solution required to get that amount.

**Method 2:** Use the V1C1=V2C2 formula. V1 is 600 mL, C1 is 25 mg/mL, V2 is unknown stock solution volume, and C2 is 100 mg/mL in this example.

To find V2, divide both sides by 1 mL/100 mL.

Because VC=AI, this strategy works (Active Ingredient). In both solutions, the AI is the same.

The total components are ten, with 2.5/10 representing a 10% solution and 7.5/10 being a 0% solution (diluent).

- Use this procedure if all of the answers are expressed in % strength; otherwise, one of the previous two ways is preferable.

The number of active ingredients and the volume of the final solution must be established to compute the final concentration of a combination of two or more solutions with differing strengths.

What is the final solution's percent strength?

- First, figure out how much active components are in each of the three solutions.
- Add the three solutions' volumes and active components together.

165 mL = 100 mL + 25 mL + 40 mL

40 g plus 22.5 g plus 30 g equals 92.5 g

- Calculate the percent strength of 92.5 g/165 mL.

# Powder Volume Calculations

Bottles or vials containing a dry powder are reconstituted with a diluent, generally water, for powder volume calculations. You can be requested to solve for the final volume, final concentration, weight of the active component, diluent volume, or powder volume, among other things. These issues may seem difficult at first look, but when broken down into smaller sections, they are not.

Each of these issues has five components in common.

- **Final Volume of the Solution (FV):** The volume of the solution after the diluent and powder have been combined, commonly measured in milliliters.
- **Powder Volume (PV):** The volume of dry powder, commonly measured in milliliters.

- **Diluent Volume (DV):** The amount of diluent (typically water) used to the dry powder to form the final solution, given in milliliters.
- **Final Concentration (FC):** After the powder and diluent have been combined, the concentration of the final solution is commonly reported in gmLor mg.
- **Active Ingredient Weight (WT):** The active ingredient's weight.

## Summary:

| Final Volume (FV) | Volume after Diluent and powder have been mixed. | If two out of these three items are known, the third can be calculated. **PV + DV = FV** |
|---|---|---|
| Powder Volume (PV) | Volume of the powder. | |
| Diluent Volume (DV) | Volume of the diluent (usually water). | |
| Final Concentration (FC) | Concentration of the solution. | If these two items are known, the FV can be calculated.<br>**(WT)(FC with mL on top) = FV Also, WT/FV = FC** |
| Weight of Active Ingredient (WT) | Weight of the active ingredient. | |

It's worth noting that not all of the issues will need all five components. The volume of the diluent would be 10 ml - 2 ml = 8 ml.

# Getting Rid of Powder Volume Issues

**Step 1:** Make a list of each of the five elements.

| Final Volume (FV) |
| --- |
| Powder Volume (PV) |
| Diluent Volume (DV) |
| Final Concentration (FC) |
| Weight of A.I. (WT) |

**Step 2:** Examine the issue and begin filling in the gaps with the data provided.

**Step 3:** Using the information provided, calculate the remaining amounts.

**Example 1: To prepare an injectable solution with a final concentration of 375 mg/mL, add 3.3 mL to a 1.5 g vial of the active component. What is the size of the powder?**

| | |
| --- | --- |
| Final Volume (FV) | |
| Powder Volume (PV) | |
| Diluent Volume (DV) | 3.3 mL |
| Final Concentration (FC) | 375 mg/mL |
| Weight of A.I. (WT) | 1.5 g |

- Calculate the final volume from the final concentration and weight of the active component after filling in the table with the information supplied in the problem.

- Finish by filling in the final volume.

| | |
|---|---|
| Final Volume (FV) | 4 mL |
| Powder Volume (PV) | |
| Diluent Volume (DV) | 3.3 mL |
| Final Concentration (FC) | 375 mg/mL |
| Weight of A.I. (WT) | 1.5 g |

- The powder volume is 0.7 mL since the final volume is 4 mL and the diluent volume is 3.3 mL.

| | |
|---|---|
| Final Volume (FV) | 4 mL |
| Powder Volume (PV) | 0.7 mL |
| Diluent Volume (DV) | 3.3 mL |
| Final Concentration (FC) | 375 mg/mL |
| Weight of A.I. (WT) | 1.5 g |

# Using Two Different Concentrations to Solve Problems

**Example 2: A 10 g vial's label states that adding 13.5 mL of diluent to the vial's contents would result in a concentration of**

When you add 9.5 mL, what concentration do you get?

**Step 1:** Complete the first section of the issue by filling in the known values.

| | |
|---|---|
| Final Volume (FV) | |
| Powder Volume (PV) | |
| Diluent Volume (DV) | 13.5 mL |
| Final Concentration (FC) | 1 g/2.5 mL |
| Weight of A.I. (WT) | 10 g |

**Step 2:** Determine the total volume.

2.5 mL 10 g 1gram Equals 25 milliliters

**Step 3:** Subtract the DV from the FV to get the Powder Volume. 11.5 mL = 25 mL - 13.5 mL

**Step 4:** Complete the last two components.

| | |
|---|---|
| Final Volume (FV) | 25 mL |
| Powder Volume (PV) | 11.5 mL |
| Diluent Volume (DV) | 13.5 mL |
| Final Concentration (FC) | 1 g/2.5 mL |
| Weight of A.I. (WT) | 10 g |

The issue now asks for the final concentration if 8.5 mL of diluent is used instead of 13.5 mL. If a different amount of diluent is supplied, the weight of the active component and the power volume will not vary.

**Step 5:** Create a second column for the second scenario and populate it with the known data.

|  | If 13.5 mL is added. | If 8.5 mL is added. |
|---|---|---|
| Final Volume | 25 mL |  |
| Powder Volume | 11.5 mL | 11.5 mL |
| Diluent Volume | 13.5 mL | 8.5 mL |
| Final Concentration | 1 g/2.5 mL |  |
| Weight of Active Ingredient | 10 g | 10 g |

In the second situation, the final volume is computed by combining the powder and diluent volumes (11.5 mL + 8.5 mL = 20 mL).

**Step 6:** Add the 20 mL computation to the second column's list.

**Step 7:** Using the weight of the active component (10 g) and the final volume, calculate the concentration of the second solution (20 mL).

|  | If 13.5 mL is added. | If 8.5 mL is added. |
|---|---|---|
| Final Volume | 25 mL | 20 mL |
| Powder Volume | 11.5 mL | 11.5 mL |
| Diluent Volume | 13.5 mL | 8.5 mL |
| Final Concentration | 1 g/2.5 mL | 1 g/2 mL |
| Weight of Active Ingredient | 10 g | 10 g |

# Chapter 6

# Miscellaneous Subjects And Exercises

**Terminology:**

- Electrolytes are ions that are essential to the body's operation. ($Na+$, $K+$, $Cl-$, and so on.)
- Ion: An atom or a collection of atoms with one or more electrons lost or gained, and a positive or negative charge.
- Cation: An ion with a positive charge (pronounced cat-ion).
- An ion with a negative charge is known as an anion.
- Valence: The quantity of charges on an ion is the simplest definition.
- Atomic Mass/Atomic Weight: These words are interchangeable for this work. They are the elements' respective weights. Hydrogen, for example, has an atomic mass of one, whereas carbon has an atomic mass of twelve. Carbon atoms are twelve times heavier than hydrogen atoms. Atomic masses do not have units.

# Understanding Milliequivalent Calculations: Key Concepts

- Measurements of ions and charges, not weights, are used in mEq computations. Not pounds of coffee beans, but dozens of eggs.
- A millimole (mmole) is equal to 1/1000 of a mole (mol), or 6.022 X 1020. • A mmol of charges is equal to one mEq.

**Examples:**

- One mol of NaCl equals one mol of Na+ and one mol of Cl-.
- Both Na+ and Cl- have a single charge.
- 1 mmol NaCl is equal to 1 mEq Na+ and 1 mEq Cl-.
- 1 mmol MgSO4 is equal to 1 mmol Mg+2 and 1 mmol SO4-2.
- There are two charges in Mg+2 and SO4-2.
- 1 mmol MgSO4 equals 2 mEq Mg+2 and 2 mEq SO4-2

## Converting from mg to mEq

- The weight and valence of a mmol of electrolyte must be known. • Calculate the weight of a mmol of an electrolyte by finding up the atomic mass and multiplying it by mg to get the mg/mmol. Potassium

(K) has an atomic mass of 39.1, which translates to 39.1 mg/mmol.

- Look up the valence to find out what it is. In the milliequivalent exercise, you'll find a list of common electrolytes and their valences.

# Temperature Conversion Calculators

Temperature conversions are carried out using a formula that varies based on the two temperature scales being compared.

To convert 50 degrees Celsius (centigrade) to Fahrenheit, for example, we use the formula below: F = 9/5 + 32 F = C * 9/5 + 32 F = C * 9/5 + 32 F

F = 50 * 9/5 + 32 F = 50 * 9/5 + 32 F = 50 *90 + 32 = F

122 = F

A temperature of 50 degrees Celsius equals 122 degrees Fahrenheit.

# Converting Temperature Scales Formulas

To convert from one temperature scale to another, use the following temperature conversion formulae.

## Celsius Temperature Conversion Formula

| Celsius to Fahrenheit Conversion | $[°F] = [°C] \times 9/5 + 32$ |
| --- | --- |
| Celsius to Kelvin Conversion | $[K] = [°C] + 273.15$ |
| Celsius to Rankine Conversion | $[°R] = [°C] \times 9/5 + 491.67$ |

## Fahrenheit Temperature Conversion Formula

| Fahrenheit to Celsius Conversion | $[°C] = ([°F] - 32) \times 5/9$ |
| --- | --- |
| Fahrenheit to Kelvin Conversion | $[K] = ([°F] + 459.67) \times 5/9$ |
| Fahrenheit to Rankine Conversion | $[°R] = [°F] + 459.67$ |

# A Final Note

This one-of-a-kind book, designed for use in an introductory pharmacy technician calculations course, covers not only the calculations that technicians will encounter in retail, but also those required for compounding, IV therapy, metrics, and other areas where a pharmacy technician may be called upon more frequently due to a shortage of pharmacists.

Furthermore, this manual employs a conversational, reader-friendly writing style as well as an easy-to-understand ratio-proportion problem-solving strategy that will aid pharmaceutical technicians to understand pharmacy calculations better and fully understand their benefit for humans.

# Chapter 7
## Exercises

## Rounding Exercises

| Rounding Exercise | | | | | |
|---|---|---|---|---|---|
| | Round to the Nearest Tenth | Rounded Number | | Round to the Nearest Hundredth | Rounded Number |
| 1 | 6.88 | 6.9 | 26 | 89.568 | 89.57 |
| 2 | 7.54 | | 27 | 45.789 | |
| 3 | 2.22 | | 28 | 1.005 | |
| 4 | 3.98 | | 28 | 2.895 | |
| 5 | 78.53 | | 30 | 3.997 | |
| 6 | 99.23 | | 31 | 7.894 | |
| 7 | 101.16 | | 32 | 3.433 | |
| 8 | 5.44 | | 33 | 2.222 | |
| 9 | 99.99 | | 34 | 1.111 | |
| 10 | 53.247 | | 35 | 8.895 | |
| 11 | 9.355 | | 36 | 3.578 | |
| 12 | 100.01 | | 37 | 2.2256 | |

| | | | | | |
|---|---|---|---|---|---|
| 13 | 56.3756 | | 38 | 90.3895 | |
| 14 | 9.56 | | 39 | 78.451 | |
| 15 | 22.56 | | 40 | 3.215 | |
| 16 | 78.59 | | 41 | 9.782 | |
| 17 | 77.459 | | 42 | 10.554 | |
| 18 | 3.57 | | 43 | 3.987 | |
| 19 | 9.78 | | 44 | 1.9954 | |
| 20 | 23.598 | | 45 | 2.493 | |
| 21 | 78.3 | | 46 | 8.523 | |

# Scientific Notation Exercise

**Convert or change the below numbers to scientific notation.**

| Number | Coefficient | # of Places from New Decimal Point to end of Original Number | Coefficient X 10 Raised to the Number of Places the Decimal Point was Moved |
|---|---|---|---|
| 67,000 | 6.7 | 4 | **6.7 X 10⁴** |
| 2,387,000 | 2.387 | 6 | **2.387 X 10⁶** |
| 7,000,000 | | | |
| 98,000 | | | |
| 432,000,000 | | | |
| 900,000,000 | | | |
| 58,000,000,000 | | | |
| 2,478,000,000 | | | |
| 92,000,000 | | | |
| 60,230,000,000 | | | |
| 105,000 | | | |

# Change the below decimal numbers to scientific notation.

| Decimal Number | Coefficient | # of Places from New Decimal Point to Original Decimal Point | Coefficient X 10 Raised to the Negative Number of Places the Decimal Point was Moved |
|---|---|---|---|
| 0.056 | 5.6 | 2 | $5.6 \times 10^{-2}$ |
| 0.000380 | 3.80 | 4 | $3.80 \times 10^{-4}$ |
| 0.00007 | | | |
| 0.00002039 | | | |
| 0.0005078 | | | |
| 0.00001832 | | | |
| 0.000650 | | | |
| 0.0000000012 | | | |
| 0.000054 | | | |
| 0.000783 | | | |
| 0.00034 | | | |

# Convert or change the below numbers from scientific notation to numbers.

| Scientific Notation | Coefficient | Exponent | # of Places to Move the Decimal Point to the Right | Number |
|---|---|---|---|---|
| $5.62 \times 10^6$ | 5.62 | 6 | 6 | 5,620,000 |
| $7.8 \times 10^7$ | 7.8 | 7 | 7 | 78,000,000 |
| $9 \times 10^5$ | | | | |
| $6.02 \times 10^7$ | | | | |
| $1.05 \times 10^4$ | | | | |
| $9.78 \times 10^9$ | | | | |
| $6.99 \times 10^3$ | | | | |
| $3.78 \times 10^8$ | | | | |
| $4.0 \times 10^8$ | | | | |
| $7.66 \times 10^5$ | | | | |

# Change or convert the below decimal numbers from scientific notation to decimal numbers.

| Scientific Notation | Coefficient | Exponent | # of Places to Move the Decimal Point to the Left | Decimal Number |
|---|---|---|---|---|
| 6.05 X 10$^{-4}$ | 6.05 | -4 | 4 | **0.000605** |
| 2.3 X 10$^{-7}$ | 2.3 | -7 | 7 | **0.00000023** |
| 7.80 X 10$^{-4}$ | | | | |
| 3.5 X 10$^{-6}$ | | | | |
| 8.995 X 10$^{-5}$ | | | | |
| 1.023 X 10$^{-9}$ | | | | |
| 5.00 X 10$^{-4}$ | | | | |

# Significant Figures Exercise

# Decide the number of significant figures in the below measurements.

| Measurement | Decimal Point? Yes or No | Yes: All Digits are Significant Except the Leading Zeros | No: All Digits are Significant Except Trailing Zeros | Number of Significant Figures |
|---|---|---|---|---|
| 605.30 cm | Yes | 605.30 cm | | 5 |
| 0.0050 cm | Yes | 0.0050 cm | | 2 |
| 905,000 mi | No | | 905,000 mi | 3 |
| 1,000,000 ft | No | | 1,000,000 ft | 1 |
| 0.00001 mi | | | | |
| 1,000,006 ft | | | | |
| 500 ft | | | | |
| 367 ft | | | | |
| 0.0051 g | | | | |
| 0.040 g | | | | |
| 92,000,000 | | | | |
| 92,000,000.0 | | | | |
| 807.01 cm | | | | |

Decide the sums or differences for the below measurements using the rules for adding and subtracting significant figures.

| Measurements | Sum or Difference Before Rounding | Least Accurate Measurement(s) | Answer Rounded to Correct Place |
|---|---|---|---|
| 7.12 mg + 6.1 mg + 7.06 mg | 20.28 mg | 6.1 mg | 20.3 mg |
| 100.5 mg + 110 mg | 210.5 mg | 110 mg | 210 mg |
| 6 cm + 8.3 cm | | | |
| 103 g + 1.1 g | | | |
| 5 ft + 52 ft | | | |
| 6.3 cm - 3 cm | | | |
| 101 mg + 25 mg | | | |
| 98.1 mg + 10 mg | | | |
| 65.5551 g + 2 g | | | |
| 1000 mi + 10 mi | | | |

Decide the products of the below measurements using the rules for multiplying and dividing significant figures.

| Measurements | Product before Rounding | Measurement with Least # of Sig Figures | Rounded Answer |
|---|---|---|---|
| 31 cm X 9 cm | 279 sq cm | 9 cm (1 sig fig) | 300 sq cm |
| 100 cm x 892 cm | 89,200 sq cm | 100 cm (1 sig fig) | 90,000 sq cm |
| 61 ft X 561 ft | | | |

# Roman Numeral Exercise

You need to be aware of the 8 basic Roman numerals and their number counterparts:  SS, I, V, X, L, C, D, M. Fill in the blanks in the following tables.

| Roman Numeral | Number | Number | Roman Numeral |
|---|---|---|---|
| SS | | 1/2 (0.5) | |
| I | | 1 | |
| V | | 5 | |
| X | | 10 | |
| L | | 50 | |
| C | | 100 | |
| D | | 500 | |
| M | | 1000 | |

**Fill in the blanks with the corresponding Roman numerals or numbers.**

| | | |
|---|---|---|
| 50 | | C |
| 100 | | 5 |
| 1/2 | | 10 |
| X | | L |
| M | | I |
| 5 | | X |
| V | | D |
| 500 | | M |
| L | | X |
| SS | | V |
| 1000 | | L |
| 1 | | C |
| D | | 5 |
| L | | 50 |

**Fill in the blanks with the corresponding Roman numerals and try not to look at the table on page 7 until you are ready to check your answers.**

| 1000 | | 100 | | 10 | | 1 | |
|------|---|-----|---|----|---|---|---|
| 2000 | | 200 | | 20 | | 2 | |
| 3000 | | 300 | | 30 | | 3 | |
| | | 400 | | 40 | | 4 | |
| | | 500 | | 50 | | 5 | |
| | | 600 | | 60 | | 6 | |
| | | 700 | | 70 | | 7 | |
| | | 800 | | 80 | | 8 | |
| | | 900 | | 90 | | 9 | |
| | | | | | | 1/2 | |

Complete the blanks with the corresponding number or Roman numeral.

| | | |
|---|---|---|
| 10 | | LXX |
| 30 | | 20 |
| 400 | | CCC |
| DC | | CD |
| 2000 | | CM |
| 8 | | 700 |
| XC | | 50 |
| 40 | | 20 |
| 60 | | LXXX |
| 200 | | DCC |
| 900 | | 600 |

**Example: Write 2782 as a Roman numeral.**
- **Line up the Roman numerals in order starting with the largest.**

  **MMDCCLXXXII**

**Example: Write MMDCLXXVI as a number.**

| MM | 2000 |
|---|---|
| DC | 600 |
| LXX | 70 |
| VI | 6 |

**Total the numbers.**

> **2676**

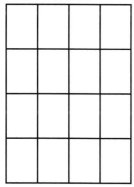

**3564 1437**

**1369 3421**

**MMDCLXVII MCMLI**

| | | | |
|---|---|---|---|
| | | | |
| | | | |
| | | | |
| | | | |

**CCCXLV DCLXII**

| | | | |
|---|---|---|---|
| | | | |
| | | | |
| | | | |

# Unit Conversion Exercise using Dimensional Analysis

| Given to be Converted | Conversion Factor (Tool) | Units of the Answer | Answer: |
|---|---|---|---|
| 3.5 g | 1000 mg/g | mg | **3500 mg** |
| 3400 g | 1 kg/1000 g | kg | **3.4 kg** |

| | | | |
|---|---|---|---|
| 25 mg | | g | |
| 8.1 kg | | lb | |
| 320 mg | | g | |
| 3 tbs | | tsp | |
| 245 cm | | m | |
| 2.2 kg | | lb | |
| 967 mcg | | mg | |
| 45 mg | | mcg | |
| 188 lb | | kg | |
| 2.5 L | | mL | |
| 502 g | | kg | |
| 89 mm | | cm | |
| 400 mL | | L | |

| | | kg | |
|---|---|---|---|
| 923 g | | | |
| 8 kg | | g | |
| 3.2 m | | cm | |
| 389 mL | | L | |

| Given to be Converted | Conversion Factor (Tool) | Units of the Answer | Answer: (Given) (Tool) |
|---|---|---|---|
| 25 mm | | cm | |
| 9.5 in | | cm | |
| 50 g | | mg | |
| 0.25 L | | mL | |
| 45 cm | | in | |
| 679 cm | | m | |
| 90 g | | kg | |

| 245 lb | | kg | |
|--------|--|----|--|

# Unit Conversion Exercise using Ratio Proportion

| Given | Units of the Answer | Set up Equation | Answer (Solve for x) |
|-------|---------------------|-----------------|----------------------|
| 3.5 g | mg | $\dfrac{x\ mg}{00\ mg}\ \dfrac{}{1\ g}$ | **3500 mg** |
| 3400 g | kg | $\dfrac{3400\ g}{x\ kg} = \dfrac{1\ kg}{1000\ g}$ | **3.4 kg** |
| 25 mg | g | | |
| 8.1 kg | lb | | |
| 320 mg | g | | |
| 3 tbs | tsp | | |
| 245 cm | m | | |
| 2.2 kg | lb | | |
| 967 mcg | mg | | |

| Given | Units of the Answer | Set up Equation | Answer (Solve for x) |
|---|---|---|---|
| 45 mg | mcg | | |
| 188 lb | kg | | |
| 2.5 L | mL | | |
| 502 g | kg | | |
| 89 mm | cm | | |
| 400 mL | L | | |
| 923 g | kg | | |
| 8 kg | g | | |
| 3.2 m | cm | | |
| 389 mL | L | | |

| | | | |
|---|---|---|---|
| 25 mm | cm | | |
| 9.5 in | cm | | |
| 50 g | mg | | |
| 0.25 L | mL | | |
| 45 cm | in | | |
| 679 cm | m | | |
| 90 g | kg | | |
| 245 lb | kg | | |

# Hours and Minutes Conversion Exercise

# Dosage Exercises Level 1

1. A patient has a prescription for a drug that comes in 500 mg/5 mL dosages. She will be given 400 mg. How much will she drink in milliliters?

2. The doctor has prescribed an 800 mg dosage. The drug comes in a 200 mg/10 mL dose. To fulfil the order, how many milliliters would be required?

3. A patient has placed a 1500 mcg prescription. 500 mcg pills are available at the drugstore. How many pills are required to complete the order?

4. A 480 mL bottle of 20% KCl is available at the drugstore. A patient's prescription states that he or she should take 15 mL per day. How many doses can this bottle provide?

5. A patient has placed an order for 14,000 heparin units. It comes in a 10 mL vial with 10,000 units/mL. What is the exact amount of milliliters required?

6. The doctor has prescribed a 65-milligram dosage. The drug comes in a 100 mg/10 mL dose. To fulfill the order, how many milliliters would be required?

7. How much mcg of levothyroxine are in two 0.125 mg levothyroxine tablets?

8. A patient has placed a 1.6 mg prescription. 0.4 mg pills are available at the drugstore. How many pills are required to complete the order?

9. A patient will be given 5 mL of medicine with a 25 mg/mL strength. How many milligrams will the patient take?

10. A prescriber has placed an order for 375 mg of medication with a 75 mg/mL strength. How many milliliters will the patient drink?

# Dosage Exercises Level 2

1. A patient is given 150 mg of medicine three times a day in three equal doses. The medication comes in 10 mL vials with a 10 mg/mL concentration. For each dosage, how many milliliters will be given?

2. A 185-pound patient will be given a daily dose of 2 mg/kg for four days. The medication comes in 10 mL vials with a 50 mg/mL concentration. How much total mL will be given out throughout the four days?

3. A patient has been prescribed 600 mg per day, divided into four equal doses. The medication comes in 10 mL vials with a 50 mg/mL concentration. In one dosage, how many mL will the patient receive?

4. A patient is given 250 mg three times a day for ten days. The medication comes in 125 mg capsules. How many pills will be given out over the 10 days?

5. For a patient weighing 80 kg, 3 mg/kg/day for 7 days is suggested. The medicine comes in 5 mL vials with a 50 mg/mL concentration. How many vials will be required throughout the seven days? Convert 3 mg/kg/day to 3 mg/kg*day as a tip.

6. A patient will be given 5 mL of medication three times every day for ten days. The medicine comes in a 240

mL container with a strength of 25 mg/mL. In each dosage, how many mg will the patient receive?

7.  A 205-pound patient is given a 600-milligram intravenous (IV) dose over two hours. The medicine comes in 10 mL vials with a concentration of 100 mg/mL. How many milliliters (mL) will be given?

8.  A patient will be given a daily dose of 34 mg/kg for 60 days. The patient is 196 pounds. The medicine comes in 20 mL vials with a 200 mg/mL concentration. For a 60-day course of treatment, how many vials will be required?

9.  A patient is given 250 mg four times a day for ten days. The medicine is available in packages of 100 250 mg capsules. How many pills will be given out throughout the 10-day therapy?

10. For 30 days, a patient is provided 1 drop in each eye twice daily. The eye drops come in a 5 mL container with 20 drops per mL. For the 30 days, how many bottles will be required?

# IV Flow Rate Calculations Exercise

**Calculate the flow rate in milliliters per hour.**

1.  A total of 1000 mL was injected over 5 hours.

2.  250 mL infusing for 2 hours

**Calculate the gtts/min flow rate. To the closest drop, turn around.**

3.  1000 mL infused over 4 hours with a drop factor of 10 (10 gtts/mL) infusion set

4.  250 mL infused over 2 hours with a drop factor of 15 using an infusion set.

5.  2 L injected over 24 hours with a drop factor of 20 using an infusion set.

6.  100 mL infused over 1 hour utilizing a drop factor of 10 infusion set

7.  1000 mL injected over 5 hours with a drop factor of 20 using an infusion set.

**Determine how long it will take to inject the following quantities.**

8.  Infusing a 1000 mL bag at a rate of 45 mL/h.

9.  A 1000 mL bag was infused at a rate of 45 mL/h with a drop factor of 20 using an infusion set.

10. A 1000 mL bag was administered at a rate of 45 mL/h with a drop factor of 10 using an infusion set.

11. A 1 L bag injected at a rate of 50 gtts/min with a drop factor of 15 using an infusion set. 12) A 500 mL bag

infused at a rate of 25 gtts/min with a drop factor of 20 using an infusion set.

**Please respond to the following questions:**

13.   A patient is prescribed regular insulin at an hourly rate of 18 units. The solution contains 100 mL of regular insulin and 100 units of regular insulin. A drop factor of 20 is employed in the infusion set. In gtts/min, what will be the flow rate?

14.   A patient is being infused with medication at a rate of 5 mcg/kg/min. The patient weighs 185 pounds and a 500 mL bag contains 250 milligrams of the medication. A drop factor of 20 is employed in the infusion set. What is the gtts/min flow rate?

15.   A patient has received a prescription for a medicine that must be administered at a rate of 25 mg/kg/h. The patient weighs 80 kg and a 1 L bag contains 10 g of the medicine. A drop factor of 15 is employed in the infusion set. What is the gtts/min flow rate?

# Percent Exercise

**Change the below numbers to percentages using the format.**

| | |
|---|---|
| 0.35 | (0.35)(100%)=35% |
| 15/17 | (15/17)(100%)=88.24% |
| 0.98 | |
| 1.78 | |
| 3.99 | |
| 0.05 | |
| 0.003 | |
| 1.25 | |
| 6/9 | |
| 5.45 | |
| 9.95 | |
| 0.005 | |

**Change the below percentages to numbers using the format.**

| | |
|---|---|
| 56% | $\frac{56\%}{100\%} = 0.56$ |
| 3.5% | |
| 99% | |
| 101% | |
| 34.5% | |
| 85.67% | |
| 3.35% | |
| 3% | |

# Percent Strength Exercise

Include the kind of solution (w/w, w/v, v/v, v/w) and express the following as a percent strength solution.

1.  200 mL KCl (7 g)

2.  1000 mL 3.5 g NaCl

3.  In 100 mL, 7.9 mg NaHCO3

4.  0.25 mL NaCl, 5 mcg

5.  3 L NaCl (45 g)

6.  200 g HC ointment with 3 g HC

7.  300 g coal tar ointment with 5 g coal tar

8.  10 g betamethasone ointment with 5 mg betamethasone

9.  urea ointment (20 g urea in 40 g urea)

10. 300 g salicylic acid cream with 18 g salicylic acid

11. 1000 mL IPA solution with 900 mL IPA

12. 40 mL ETOH in a solution of 100 mL ETOH

**Please respond to the following questions:**

13. In 10 mL of 0.9 percent NaCl (normal saline), how many mg of NaCl are there?

14. How much sodium chloride (NaCl) is in 2 liters of NS (normal saline)?

15. In 473 mL of 20% KCl, how many g of KCl are there?

16. In 30 mL of 0.5 percent bupivacaine solution, how many mg of bupivacaine are there?

17. In 100 mL of 1% lidocaine, how many mg of lidocaine are there?

18. If there are 20 drops/mL, how many mcg of NaCl are in one drop of 0.9 percent NaCl?

19. In 60 mL of 80 proof (40 percent ETOH) tequila, how many mL of ETOH are there?

20. In 500 g of 2.5 percent HC ointment, how many grams of HC are there?

# Percent Error Exercise

1. **The preferred volume is 46 mL, but you measured out 48 mL.**

| Desired Quantity (Target) | Actual Quantity | Error Quantity | Percent Error |
|---|---|---|---|
|  |  |  |  |

2. **The preferred weight is 350 mg, the main weight is 376 mg.**

| Desired Quantity (Target) | Actual Quantity | Error Quantity | Percent Error |
|---|---|---|---|
|  |  |  |  |

3.  **The preferred volume is 2.3 L, but the actual volume is 2.2 L.**

| Desired Quantity (Target) | Actual Quantity | Error Quantity | Percent Error |
|---|---|---|---|
|  |  |  |  |

4.  **The preferred weight is 2.5 kg, but the main weight is 1.7 kg.**

| Desired Quantity (Target) | Actual Quantity | Error Quantity | Percent Error |
|---|---|---|---|
|  |  |  |  |

5.  **The preferred weight is 7.4 g, but the actual weight is 6.8 g.**

| Desired Quantity (Target) | Actual Quantity | Error Quantity | Percent Error |
|---|---|---|---|
|  |  |  |  |

# Ratio Strength Exercises

1.  In 500 mL of a 1:10,000 solution, how many grams of an active component are there?

2.  In 40 mL of a 1:200 solution, how many grams of an active component are there?

3.  In 600 g of a 1:25 w/w preparation, how many grams of an active component are there?

4. In 800 mL of a 1:10,000 solution, how many milligrams of an active component are there?

5. In 10 mL of a 1:100,000 solution, how many mcg are there?

6. You've been given a 10 mL vial labeled 1:10,000 and told to draw up 0.4 mg of medication. How many milliliters (mL) would you draw?

7. You need to prepare 200 g of a 1:100 HC ointment. How much HC powder would you use, and how much ointment base would you use?

8. You have a solution with a concentration of 1:10,000 w/v. What is the strength as a percentage?

9. What is the strength of a 1:100 w/v solution in percentages?

10. You have a 100 mL vial with a 1:1000 label. How many milligrams are there in a 25 mL solution?

## Concentrations and Dilutions Exercise

1. A customer requests 600 mL of a 17 percent solution. You have a 43 percent solution in your possession. How many milliliters of stock solution (43 percent) and milliliters of diluent are required?

2. A 35 percent solution is available at the drugstore. A doctor issues a prescription for 40 milliliters of 250 milliliters-per-milliliter solution. How many milliliters of stock solution and milliliters of diluent is required? Even if the concentrations of the two solutions are not in the same units, you may apply V1C1=V2C2. It's worth a shot.

3. A prescription for 300 mL of a 16 percent solution is written. In the drugstore, you may get a 50 percent solution. How many milliliters of stock solution and milliliters of diluent is required?

4. A prescription for 60 mL of a 50 mg/mL solution is brought in by a patient. A 360 mg/2 mL solution is available at your drugstore. How many milliliters of stock solution and milliliters of diluent is required?

5. Your pharmacy has a 150 mL 1:1000 stock bottle and a 200 mL stock bottle of the same medicine in an 8% solution. The pharmacist, for no apparent reason other than to make your life harder, mixes the two bottles together and instructs you to create 300 mL of a 30 mg/mL solution. How many milliliters of mixed stock solution and milliliters of diluent is required?

6. The pharmacist has both a 15% and a 75% alcohol solution on hand. A prescription for 300 mL of a 40% alcohol solution is written for you. How many milli-

liters of each of the 15% and 75% solutions are required?

7.   An order for 700 mL of a 34 percent solution is placed. Your pharmacy has both a 10% and a 45 percent solution on hand. How many milliliters of each of the 10% and 45% solutions are required?

8.   What is the percentage strength of a solution that contains 60 mL of a 10% solution and 180 mL of a 35% solution?

9.   Combine D10W and D40W to make 200 mL of 19 percent dextrose solution. What is the exact amount of each? (Note that D10W is 10% dextrose in water and D40W equals 40% dextrose in water.)

10.  In issue 5, the same pharmacist combines 100 mL of a 6% solution, 200 mL of a 100 mg/mL solution, and 1 L of a 1:100 solution, then takes 10 mL of that combination and mixes it with 120 mL of diluent. What is the final solution's percent strength?

# Powder Volume Calculations

| Final Volume (FV) | Volume after Diluent and powder have been mixed. | If two out of these three items are known, the third can be calculated. **PV + DV = FV** |
|---|---|---|
| Powder Volume (PV) | Volume of the powder. | |
| Diluent Volume (DV) | Volume of the diluent (usually water). | |
| Final Concentration (FC) | Concentration of the solution. | If these two items are known, the FV can be calculated. |
| Weight of Active Ingredient (WT) | Weight of the active ingredient. | **(WT)(FC with mL on top) = FV Also, WT/FV = FC** |

Draw a container with the powder at the bottom and the diluent on top of the powder in this area. Label the final volume with a bracket that includes the powder and the diluent. Make a few dots in the powder to symbolize genuine medicine. (The powder frequently contains fillers and other ingredients that aren't genuine medicine.) The dots will indicate the real drug's weight.

1. **A vial's label specifies that it holds 3 g. It also states that you should add 15.3 mL to create the solution 100 mg/mL. What is the size of the powder?**

Final Volume (FV)

_____

Powder Volume (PV)

_____

Diluent Volume (DV)

_____

Final Concentration (FC)

_____

Weight of A.I. (WT)

2. A reconstituted gastric suspension will have a dosage of 250 mg/5 mL. With a powder volume of 14.9 mL, the A.I. is 5 g. How much water do you need to add?

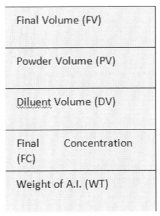

| |
|---|
| Final Volume (FV) |
| Powder Volume (PV) |
| Diluent Volume (DV) |
| Final Concentration (FC) |
| Weight of A.I. (WT) |

3. A container of amoxicillin instructs you to add 187 mL to create a 125 mg/5 mL suspension. The amoxicillin in the bottle is 5 g. What is the size of the powder?

| |
|---|
| Final Volume (FV) |
| Powder Volume (PV) |
| Diluent Volume (DV) |
| Final Concentration (FC) |
| Weight of A.I. (WT) |

# Serial Dilution Exercise

Any dilution in which the concentration declines by the same factor in each succeeding stage is referred to as a serial dilution. You double the dilution factors at each stage in serial dilutions. The original volume divided by the final volume is the dilution factor or dilution.

DF=ViVf

For example, to make 10 mL of solution, mix a 1 mL sample with 9 mL of diluent.

DF=ViVf = 1mL10mL=110. This is a 1:10 dilution.

**Example 1:**

**When you add 0.2 mL of a stock solution to 3.8 mL of diluent, what is the dilution factor?**

Vf = 0.2 mL + 3.8 mL = 4.0 mL

DF=ViVf = 0.2mL4.0mL=120. This is a 1:20 dilution.
**Example No. 2**

**What would the ultimate dilution factor be if you repeated the aforementioned dilution four times?**

**Solution**

Remember that serial dilutions are always done by adding a fixed amount of the original dilution to tubes of the same volume one after the other. So you double the dilution factor by each consecutive dilution.

Mix 0.2 mL of diluent from Tube 1 with 3.8 mL of diluent from Tube 2. Then, in Tube 3, add 0.2 mL of diluent to 3.8 mL of diluent and stir. Rep this step till you have four tubes.

After four dilutions, the dilution factor is:

DF=120×120×120×120=1160000 = 1:160 000

Tube 4's concentration would be 100 g/L if the original stock solution's concentration was 100 g/L.

$100 \ \mu g/\mu L \times 1160000 = 6.25 \times 10^{-4} \ \mu g/\mu L$

# Miliequivalent Calculations Exercise

| Name | Atomic Symbol | Atomic Mass | Ionic Form |
|---|---|---|---|
| Hydrogen | H | | H·(Hydrogen Ion) |
| Carbon | C | | |
| Oxygen | O | | |
| Sodium | Na | | Na·(Sodium Ion) |
| Magnesium | Mg | | Mg⁺⁺(Magnesium Ion) |
| Chlorine | Cl | | Cl·(Chloride Ion) |
| Potassium | K | | K·(Potassium Ion) |
| Calcium | Ca | | Ca⁺⁺(Calcium Ion) |
| Sulfur | S | | |

1.    Determine the atomic masses of the following elements. The atomic masses can be found on the

periodic table or by doing an online search. If you can't find anything on your own, they're mentioned in the answers. To the fraction of a percent, round up.

2.    So now you understand the atomic masses of each element, enter in the formula masses of the following polyatomic ions. Combine all of the distinct masses. CH3COO- is made up of 2 carbon atoms, three hydrogen atoms, and two oxygen atoms.

| Name | Chemical Formula | Formula Mass | Ionic Form |
|------|------------------|--------------|------------|
| Acetate | $CH_3COO^-$ | | $CH_3COO$ |
| Bicarbonate | $HCO_3-$ | | $HCO_3-$ |
| Sulfate | $SO_4-2$ | | $SO_4-2$ |

3.    You can now list the formula masses of the ionic compounds below since you've learned the atomic and formula masses.

| Name | Chemical Formula | Formula Mass | Ionic Form |
|------|------------------|--------------|------------|
| Sodium Chloride | $NaCl$ | | $Na·Cl$ |
| Potassium Chloride | $KCl$ | | $K·Cl$ |
| Calcium Chloride | $CaCl_2$ | | $Ca·2Cl$ |
| Magnesium Chloride | $MgCl_2$ | | $Mg·2Cl$ |
| Sodium Acetate | $CH_3COONa$ | | $Na·CH_3COO$ |
| Potassium Acetate | $CH_3COOK$ | | $K·CH_3COO$ |
| Magnesium Sulfate | $MgSO_4$ | | $Mg·SO_42-$ |
| Sodium Bicarbonate | $NaHCO_3$ | | $Na·HCO_3-$ |

4.  For each component, fill in the table with the mg/mmol and mEq/mmol ratios.

| Name | Chemical Formula | mg/mmol (ratio) | mEq/mmol (ratio) |
|---|---|---|---|
| Sodium Chloride | NaCl | | |
| Potassium Chloride | KCl | | |
| Calcium Chloride | $CaCl_2$ | | |
| Magnesium Chloride | $MgCl_2$ | | |
| Sodium Acetate | $CH_3COONa$ | | |
| Potassium Acetate | $CH_3COOK$ | | |
| Magnesium Sulfate | $MgSO_4$ | | |
| Sodium Bicarbonate | $NaHCO_3$ | | |

- You now have all of the necessary conversion ratios to convert between mg and mEq. For instance, how much mEq are there in 500 mg of CaCl2?
- Calcium chloride has a molecular weight of 111 mg/mol and two mEq/mol.
- You can write these ratios as 111 mg. 1 mmol
- 2 mEq and 111 mg
- 1 mol or mmol mEq = mEq = mEq = mEq

Begin by stating the issue and the units of the solution.

- mEq = 500 mg
- Fill in the ratios as normal, leaving just the answer's units blank.

**Please respond to the following questions.**

5.    In 746 mg of KCl, how many mEq are there?

6.    In 2 g of calcium chloride, how many mEq of calcium chloride are there?

7.    In 2 g of calcium chloride, how many mEq of Ca++ are there?

8.    In 10 mEq of magnesium sulfate, how many mg of magnesium sulfate are there? 9) In 12 mEq of sodium acetate, how many g of sodium acetate are there?

10.   In 2 L of 0.9 percent NaCl, how many mEq of NaCl are there?

11.   In 30 mL of 10% KCl solution, how many mEq of KCl are there?

12.   In 10 g of MgSO4, how many mEq of MgSO4 are there?

13.   In 1.5 L of 10% NaCl, how many mg of Na+ (simply sodium) are present?

14.   If you're feeling adventurous, try this one. Your buddy has 1.5 L of MgSO4 solution and you have 2.5 L of 10% NaCl solution. You have twice as much mEq NaCl as your buddy has MgSO4 mEq. What is your friend's MgSO4 % strength?

# About the Author

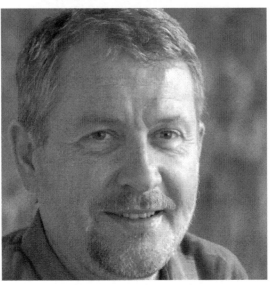

Clement Carter has a degree in Pharmacy from one of the top universities in Texas and ever since then, he has gone on to grow his pharmaceutical skills and abilities. He works as a clinical pharmacist and coaches numerous intending pharmacists who are aspiring to be the best in this field.

Clement is also a member of the American Society of Pharmacists. He lives in Arlington, Texas with his wife and three daughters.

Made in United States
Orlando, FL
10 July 2022

19609917R00061